A Piece of
Cake

A Piece of
Cake

A Remarkable Experience

R O G E R K O H L E R

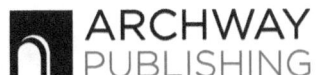
ARCHWAY
PUBLISHING

Archway Publishing books may be ordered through booksellers or by contacting:

Archway Publishing
1663 Liberty Drive
Bloomington, IN 47403
www.archwaypublishing.com
1-(888)-242-5904

Cover Photo by Nancy Bray.

Because of the dynamic nature of the Internet, any web addresses or links contained in this book may have changed since publication and may no longer be valid. The views expressed in this work are solely those of the author and do not necessarily reflect the views of the publisher, and the publisher hereby disclaims any responsibility for them.

Any people depicted in stock imagery provided by Thinkstock are models, and such images are being used for illustrative purposes only.

Certain stock imagery © Thinkstock.

ISBN: 978-1-4808-0038-0 (sc)
ISBN: 978-1-4808-0039-7 (e)

Library of Congress Control Number: 2013904589

Printed in the United States of America
Archway Publishing rev. date: 03/19/2013

To Adele

Table of Contents

Foreword

Mr. Kohler's experience was typical, but the lens through which it was seen is truly unique.

Cardiovascular disease, including coronary heart disease, valvular heart disease, strokes and rhythm abnormalities among many other facets, is remarkably prevalent in the industrialized world but remains un-diagnosed in many cases. The symptoms of cardiovascular disease can be so subtle as to elude our normal triggers of concern, and this often manifests as late presentations. Doctors and surgeons work endlessly to identify those at risk, but it is not uncommon that someone's advanced cardiovascular illness will not be identified until later stages, where intervention can be more complex.

Intimidating though they may seem, doctors are a tremendous resource for the patients they serve, and while symptoms may seem minor, they should be evaluated. More often than not, vague symptoms such as weakness or fatigue are not related to the heart, but a history, physical exam and objective testing can help determine this.

In Mr. Kohler's case, his valvular heart disease had likely been present for many years, maybe decades before an astute and wise physician in Harwich detected his murmur and likely saved his life, along with his surgeon in Boston who performed the skillful, artful and wildly complex procedure. I had the privilege of serving between these two physicians, which offered great perspective. In the end, it was Mr. Kohler whose strength and perseverance won the day. It must have been quite daunting to hear a young physician, having met his new patient only minutes before, announce that he needed a referral to a surgeon for open heart surgery. Once the initial shock and skepticism had worn away, Mr. Kohler handled his challenge with aplomb, which is why he enjoyed such a successful procedure and recovery. For him, it truly was a "Piece of Cake".

—John A. Kalin MD

Preface

I was heading for a heart attack and didn't know it.

The only sign was feeling a little tired and thinking it was normal.

I had a very thorough and astute doctor who suggested I see a cardiologist.

I had an echocardiogram and found I needed urgent open-heart surgery.

Heart Disease is the number-one killer in America today, according to the American Heart Association.

An estimated 1.1 million Americans will have a heart attack this year, and one-third of them will die.

Nearly half those who die from heart attack never showed prior symptoms of heart disease.

I wrote this story because of the extraordinary difference I felt between before and after my open-heart surgery. I was compelled to write it, and it was a great pastime during my recovery. I decided to tell the story, and if it saves one life, it will have been worth it.

Read this book—it could save your life !!!

Annual Visit

I live on Cape Cod and enjoy walking with my wife, Adele, and our golden retriever, Bella, on the many beautiful beaches we have here. I had noticed during the last six months that it was becoming more of an effort to walk the distance I'd walked easily only a short time before. I now believe I was heading for a heart attack and didn't know it, and I can imagine there are thousands of folks out there who are in the same predicament.

"Roger, have you ever seen a cardiologist?" asked Dr. Reagan, my primary care doctor.

"Me? Are you kidding? No, I have never had any chest pains, nausea, dizziness, numbness, or anything related to symptoms of a heart attack."

"I think I'll arrange for you to see a cardiologist," he said.

It was another beautiful sunny morning on Cape Cod, a day to be happy and thankful to be alive. I had gone for my yearly check up, and all looked good.

"Doctor, I feel good, but I do feel very tired sometimes."

The good doctor listened to my chest again with his stethoscope and said, "You know, I can hear a murmur. I'm going to send you to see Dr. Kalin; he is a cardiologist in Hyannis."

I drove home, and of course Adele asked how it went.

"Oh, it went great. I'm in good shape ... but Dr. Reagan has arranged for me to see a cardiologist."

"Really? Why?"

"He is just being his usual thorough self."

A few days later I got a call from Dr. Kalin's office for an appointment. I was to have an echocardiogram.

Surprise

A week later I drove twenty minutes from Harwich to Hyannis. I checked in at the counter. The receptionist said, "Please take a seat. Doctor Kalin will be with you shortly."

The assistant arrived in a few minutes, and I was shown into a room. The nurse came in to do the procedure, along with another young woman whom he introduced as a student. "Do you mind if this young lady looks on?"

"No, not at all."

I was asked to strip to my underpants and lay on a table, on my side. He proceeded to put an oily sensor over my body and around the heart area. He sat with the student and watched a screen.

I snoozed (as I did a lot then) for about forty minutes while they chatted and watched the screen, which had weird, gurgling sounds coming from it. Gurgle, whoosh, gush, gurgle, gurgle, gush, gurgle, gurgle.

He said, "Okay, that will do—we are done." He then said Dr. Kalin would be in touch.

A day later I received a call from Dr. Reagan. "Roger, I have the results from the echocardiogram and the cardiologist. Your aortic valve is not operating efficiently, which means a large portion of your blood is being pumped upward and then dropping back into the heart again, instead of going to the aorta. It means your heart is working overtime. Also there is an aneurysm forming on the root of your aorta."

"What does this mean?" I asked, concerned.

"It means your aorta is ballooning, and walls of the aorta are getting thinner. If it continues, the vessel could burst, and then you are in big trouble."

A few days later I received a call from Dr. Kalin's office, asking me to come and see him. We drove to Hyannis, parked in the parking lot, and went to the front desk. "Please take a seat, and Dr. Kalin will be with you shortly."

A nurse came, took me to a room, and proceeded to take my blood pressure and do an EKG.

When Dr. Kalin came into the room, he told me, "Roger, you need open-heart surgery and soon."

"Really? I am shocked!"

He proceeded to tell me what Dr. Reagan had said: if I did not have the surgery, my heart would enlarge, and that would not be good. "I know you don't know me, and you may think I look young to be telling you this, but you need this surgery."

I said, "What if I don't do this?"

He said, I'll give you twenty-four months or twenty-four years to live, but I don't know which." I know it may be a shock to you, and this is major surgery, but these days it goes fairly smoothly. The mortality rate is about 2 percent, or 5 percent if you are a diabetic."

I was still a little shocked. "When do you think I should have this done?"

"I think within a few weeks. I would not leave it for two years. Get a second opinion if you wish, but I know I am right. If you want to go ahead, I suggest the Beth Israel Medical Center in Boston, and I recommend the head surgeon there, Dr. Khabbaz. He is the best for this particular procedure. It is called the Bentall Procedure."

By this time it was becoming a reality for me. Whoa!

He suggested I get a CT scan, which would show even more evidence if this operation was necessary, and then I should go see Dr. Khabbaz for his assessment.

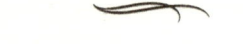

Dr. Kalin's office made an appointment for me at the Cape Cod Hospital to have the CT scan. I drove to the hospital in Hyannis, was directed to the CT scan office, and then taken to the room housing the big white machine.

A few days later I got a call from Dr. Khabbaz's office, asking me to come and see him. We set the GPS for his office at the Beth Israel Medical Center and drove the two hours from the Cape. We found the parking garage with ease and walked into Dr. Khabbaz's office next door. We checked in at the front desk and were asked to sit in the waiting room. There were two other couples there, and they looked as though they were there to see the doctor after the surgery. They were smiling, and I felt that was a good sign.

An assistant, Brooks, took us to a room and proceeded to tell me what the problem was. As before, I was told I needed a new valve and grafting work on the root of my aorta in my heart. The CT scan showed even more evidence that I was in need of surgery.

He described the two different types of valve replacement option procedures. One type was the fiber or pig valve, and the other was the mechanical valve.

At this point Dr. Khabbaz entered the room and introduced himself. He sat in chair opposite me, looked me straight in the eyes, and said, "Roger, You need this operation—and soon. You are sixty-six, and I recommend the mechanical valve. Here is the reason why. The fiber valve can last ten or fifteen years, but the mechanical valve may last forty years. If you were seventy, I would recommend the fiber valve.

If you are sixty-six and have the fiber valve, and you require the surgery again at eighty, then it can be dangerous."

He paused before continuing. "There are two drawbacks if you go with the mechanical valve. First, the operating valve makes a clicking sound, which can be heard. Most patients find it acceptable because it is a white noise and, it seems to disappear when they tune it out. Second, you have to take a blood thinner for the rest of your life. This can annoy some people because they have to have their blood checked once a month, to ensure they take the correct amount of blood thinner medication. This means once a month, you have to drive to the clinic and have a blood sample taken."

I said, "The first drawback worries me a little, because I like peace and quiet, and the noise might drive me crazy."

"No, I don't think it will worry you, because it is a white noise that seems to disappear," he said. "Some people even find the noise comforting."

"Okay, let me think about that one."

"With Coumadin, the blood thinner, there are two pages to read regarding how it works and the side effects. Read it now and tell us what you think."

I read the two pages and said, "Okay, I don't think that is going to worry me. I don't think it is a problem to go get my blood taken once a month."

They told me some people don't want to take blood thinner for another reason, and that was sports. "It can be dangerous if you are a downhill skier or want to play football, skydive, or do other sports where you could have serious injury. Having thin blood makes it more difficult for your blood to coagulate."

I said, "I'm not worried about this, because I have been skydiving twice and skied for twenty-five years, and I'm done with football, so these things are off my bucket list."

Dr. Khabbaz then told me the next step would be to have an angiogram done, which would show the condition of my arteries and whether or not I would need to have bypass surgery at the same time. They liked to know this before they started, so they did not get any rude shocks when they opened up the chest.

"I guess this is a major shock to me that I need open-heart surgery, but let me think about it."

I phoned a family friend, Gene, who'd had the same surgery a few months before. "Roger, it is A PIECE OF CAKE" he said. Gene is eighty-eight, and three months after the surgery, he went back to work three days a week.

A few days later Adele and I went to see Gene and Queenie at Pinehills, in Plymouth. We had tea and talked, and I told him my predicament.

He told me how smoothly it all went and said, "What are you waiting for, Roger?"

Gene said his heart surgeon had said he liked playing golf and had always wanted to have a couple rounds at Pinehills, where Gene and Queenie lived. Gene had said, "If I pull through this surgery, I will treat you to two rounds and dinner at the Pinehills Country Club."

The surgeon had said, "Gene, you can start writing the check now!"

Gene's comment of a piece of cake referred to how it was for the patient. We both agreed that the doctors, nurses, and assistants who performed these surgeries were to be greatly admired for performing this potentially danger-ous operation with such a high level of skill and with all the latest equipment, knowledge, and techniques. Not so many years ago, it was a life or death surgery, and now it usually went incredibly well.

We left Gene and Queenie's home at Pinehills and went for dinner at the East Bay Grill in Plymouth. Adele had cod and salad, and I had steak and salad.

I rang Dr. Kalin again and said, "Doctor, are you sure I need this surgery?"

He said. "I am 100 percent sure, but get a second opinion if you like."

I called around and made a fairly weak attempt at getting a second opinion, because I was so impressed with how definite both Dr. Kalin and Dr. Khabbaz had been.

A few days later, Dr. Kalin's office phoned to say that we should get an angiogram, which would show what shape my arteries were in. This procedure could be done at Cape Cod Hospital. They wanted to know this so that they could be prepared to do this work when they opened my chest.

They made an appointment for me, and off I went early one morning to Hyannis for this procedure, which would not only show my arteries condition but again confirm that I needed the surgery.

Adele drove me there and dropped me at the main entrance of Cape Cod Hospital. She was going to return about seven hours later to pick me up. This was necessary because the patient was not permitted to drive home.

They gave a form of local anesthetic for the procedure. It is a procedure where they put a tube into your groin and then send a dye up through your arteries and a camera to check if your arteries are blocked or partially blocked. This is a seven-hour procedure from start to finish, and they sedate you so that you are half out of it.

I walked in at the main entrance and asked at the front desk where I should go. A nurse directed me to a room, where I was given a robe and asked to undress and put on the robe. I was then taken to a bed. A short time later a nurse arrived to shave the area where the tube was to be inserted. She briefly explained the procedure. The doctor then came by to tell me what he would be doing. They gave me a shot of something in the arm and a short time later wheeled me into the operating room.

I can only vaguely recall them working on an area on the right of my groin and consulting a screen. I had to rest for a period of time after the procedure and then dress. They put me in a wheelchair and wheeled me from an area adjacent to the operating room down to the front door of the hospital, where my wife was waiting to pick me up and drive back home.

As we approached the front door of the hospital, I was wheeled past a friend of mine.

"Hey, Roger, what's up?"

"Hi, Guy. I'm doing fine. Talk to you soon."

We drove back to Harwich.

Open Heart Surgery

By this time I had decided I would definitely go ahead with the open-heart surgery, and I was dealing with the best cardiologist and heart surgeon around. The only question was whether I should go for the pig valve or the metal valve.

I rang Dr. Reagan to say I was definitely going ahead, and I asked his opinion about the valve.

"Get the metal valve. Here is the question: do you want to live another ten years and have the surgery again, or do you want to maybe go for forty years with no more surgery?"

The latter sounded better. This was now three doctors saying to go metal.

Now it was off to the dentist.

Dr. Khabbaz's office said, "We need clearance from your dentist saying that your teeth are in good shape. They have to clean your teeth and make sure you have as little bacteria in your mouth as possible."

I called my dentist. "Hi, Sue, can you please give me an appointment with Dr. Rivers?"

"So, Justin, what do you think about the metal valve?"

"Listen, buddy, no question about it. Most definitely you should get the mechanical valve. Believe me, you are going to feel great."

The count was now four to zero.

My brother in law, Anan, called to give me his assurance. He believed all would go well. The word was now out about my upcoming surgery.

"Roger, give my uncle Jay a call; he would love to talk to you about it, and after all, he is a cardiologist."

I rang Jay. He told me,

"Roger, you need the metal valve, and don't worry about people that say they can hear it clicking. It is not a problem."

Gosh, this was reassuring. Now it was five to zero.

I rang Dr. Khabbaz's office and said I would like to make an appointment for the surgery, and I would like to schedule it as soon as possible.

Two minutes later Lisa said, "Let's see, how about November 19?"

"Sounds good to me."

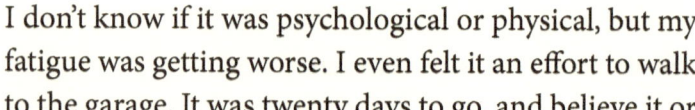

I don't know if it was psychological or physical, but my fatigue was getting worse. I even felt it an effort to walk to the garage. It was twenty days to go, and believe it or not, I started counting down the days.

It was now a reality, I was going to have open-heart surgery, and something I would never have imagined only four weeks before was going to happen.

I wondered what could have caused this. It may have been because I used to smoke twenty-five years before, or because I had rheumatic fever as a child. It may simply be genetics. However, now I just wanted to get it over and done with.

Doctor Reagan was very thorough and suggested I also see a kidney doctor in Hyannis, to check whether my kidneys were in good shape. They liked to check everything to be sure I would have a good recovery after the surgery. Dr. Reagan had detected some protein in my urine sample, and this raised some possible red flags. I drove to Hyannis and was sitting in the small office waiting to see the doctor. Another patient came in and sat opposite me. He was carrying a plastic bag with about twenty-five medications in it. The poor man looked like a traveling pharmacy.

"Mr. Kohler, please come in." The doctor told me she had looked at the results of a test and was pleased to announce my kidneys were in good shape.

That was music to my ears. I said to her, "I have been told for about the last twenty years I should drink six glasses of water a day."

She said, "I hear this all the time. It is an old wives' tale. It is important to drink plenty of fluids, but really, water does very little for your kidneys."

A couple of days later Lisa rang from Dr Khabbaz's office and gave me a time to come in for a chest X-ray; book into the hospital; meet the anesthesiologist and two assistants to Dr. Khabbaz, Dr. Courtney, and Dr. Allison; and to go through the procedure for the day of surgery.

That day Adele had appointments, so I drove myself into the hospital to register and see the doctors. I left Harwich and drove the two hours to Boston. I parked in the parking garage and walked the short distance to Beth Israel Medical Center. The front desk directed me to the fifth floor.

First I met the anesthesiologist, and she asked me all the questions one would expect to hear from an anesthesiologist.

She asked if I had any comments. "Yes: please don't let me wake up."

"You mean during the surgery?" she asked.

"Yes, of course."

She said, "Don't worry, I will make sure you wake up at the right time."

She told me I was to arrive at 6:00 a.m. on the day of the surgery wearing some comfortable clothes. I should bring nothing else with me and should register at the front main entrance of the hospital. They would then take me to the seventh floor, where they would prepare me for the surgery before wheeling me in for all the fun at 7:15 a.m.

I was then taken to another room for a chest X-ray before I headed to another room to meet the two surgeon's assistants, Dr. Courtney and Dr. Allison. We chatted, and they made me feel very comfortable and gave me great encouragement. They told me the results from the angiogram showed I would not need bypass surgery because my arteries were in good shape. I was told the surgery would take about four hours, and I would be in the intensive care unit for about three days and on the floor below that for two days.

"Wow, I will be out of there in five days? Amazing! You have made me very confident."

"Good! Do you have any questions? "

I thought I would ask one more time about Coumadin. You see, when you read about taking the blood thinner, it can freak you out. For example you may get gangrene and lose a limb or two. This is an extremely rare side effect.

After assuring me about the Coumadin, they confirmed again, "If I were you, I would go for the metal valve."

He said if it was him, he would opt for the pig valve because he loved skiing down a mountain at a hundred miles per hour, but because I had said I was finished with that, I should get the mechanical valve. He mentioned a patient who had the pig valve at age twenty-six, and now she was thirty-six and had to have the surgery again.

"Gosh, what a drag!" I decided to make it official. "I'll have the mechanical valve, please." Then I paused before I said, "I have one other question, and I hope you don't think I am rude. Is this hospital as good as the Brigham's Woman's Hospital?"

Dr. Courtney said, "I get asked this question all the time. Brigham's is a very good, big hospital, and this is a very good, small hospital."

I said, "That sounds good to me. I'll see you on the nineteenth!"

Preparation

I wanted to get this thing over and done with, and I was now really counting the days.

About a week before the nineteenth, Tina rang from Dr. Khabbaz's office. "Roger, we were wondering if you minded if we rescheduled you to the twentieth. We have an emergency."

"Oh boy ... No, of course not."

"Good, thank you. We will see you on the twentieth!"

My brother-in-law, Ronnie, and his wife, Julie, rang me to give me their best wishes, which I greatly appreciated. The time was ticking away slowly and I started to wonder, *What if this thing does not go according to plan?*

I decided to go away for a few days to pass the time, and one thing I loved doing was going to New York City and wandering around the museums. I drove to the Park and Ride at Framingham and jumped on the Limoliner, a very comfortable coach that leaves three times a day from Boston to New York. It drops people at the Hilton on Sixth Avenue.

I stayed at the Hilton for three days and visited the American Museum of National History, which I had been to before, but it was a great place to wander around for hours. I wandered among dinosaurs and fossils and the huge number of showcases of different peoples throughout time. I pondered how the dinosaurs were on the planet for a hundred million years, and humans had been here for sixty thousand years. Some writers were already predicting our demise had already started. I suddenly realized that my demise had a 2 percent chance of occurring in six days.

One night for dinner, I went to Rue Seventy-Three Restaurant, on the corner of Sixth Avenue and Seventy-third Street. It is one of those Manhattan restaurants where the food is good and is reasonably priced. Its walls are adorned with pictures of actors and celebrities from the forties, fifties, and sixties. A waitress with a gorgeous face and short cropped hair served me. I said, "I don't suppose they would like my photo for the wall." She just looked at me with a big smile on her face.

I returned to Boston on the Limoliner and waited patiently until the big day.

On the morning of the twentieth, Adele and I woke by alarm at 3:00 a.m., and I showered with special antibacterial soap. With no food in my stomach since midnight, we set off at 4:00 for the Beth Israel Medical Center in Boston.

There was no traffic, so the trip was quick. We arrived at 6:00 a.m., and I booked in.

They whisked me off to the seventh floor for surgery preparation.

Adele was taken to a waiting room that had sofas, television, and Internet connection—all the comforts for a stay of several hours.

I was taken to a room with four other folks; they were also in for surgeries the same day. We all looked at each other and smiled without much chatter. A nurse came to collect me, and I was taken to a bed where I was given a robe to change into. My clothes, which were all I had with me, were put into a bag and sent somewhere. I knew they supplied me with anything I needed in the way of toothbrush and toiletries. Adele appeared at the end of my bed. She spent a few minutes with me to give me her love and best wishes. She was then taken back to the waiting area.

I had a string of people come and introduce themselves: nurses, doctor assistants, and anesthesiologist assistants. A cheerful nurse arrived to shave my chest and arms. The anesthesiologist assistant said with a big smile on his face, "Don't you worry, we will take good care of you." The whole team continually gave me encouragement.

A young doctor arrived, and after giving me a shot of something, he proceeded to place tubes in my arms and neck. He said, "I think you know my father, Tom Jones. He is a realtor on the Cape."

"Oh, really? Yes, I do," I replied. Small world!

Shortly after they put the tube in my neck, which is used for providing medication and sedation during surgery, I vaguely remember being wheeled off to the operating room. The time was around 7:30 a.m.

I remember them putting a rubber mask over my mouth and nose.

Goodnight, Nurse …

Beth Israel

The next thing I recall was seeing something vaguely through my squinting eyes. They had closed my chest at 11:30 a.m.; I saw this on a white board later in my room. It was now around 3:00 p.m. I believe they took out the breathing tubes at this time. Adele said I was slowly waking between three and five.

I heard, "He's awake." My first view was of my beautiful wife and two nurses, whose names I later learned were Carol and Donna.

Everyone seemed to be cheering me on. I remember saying, "This is one great hospital."

My poor wife had risen that day at 3:00 a.m. and was sitting around all day until 5:00 p.m. I knew she would be exhausted and missing our dog. I said, "Please go home, pick up Bella, and have a big sleep. I'm fine."

Adele had been sitting in the room where patients' family waited for news about the surgery. She left the room to visit the bathroom, and at that time a nurse came to get her because I was waking up. When she returned, the people in the room told her that the nurse had come to get her. At that precise moment they heard from the room through the doors, "Blue Alert," which was a call when someone's feet went blue. Of course she thought it was me, and she panicked. Fortunately she learned seconds later it wasn't me. She was brought to my bed, and I believe I woke a short time later.

At 6:00 p.m. Dr. Khabbaz rang Adele and gave her the report of how the surgery had gone. What he'd expected to do before they started was to replace the aortic valve with a mechanical valve and do some grafting on the root of the aorta. When he had opened my chest, he found the aorta in better condition than expected and decided that the work on the root of it was not necessary. This was great for me because that work took longer to do and had a longer recovery. He said he thought it all went very well. I learned four weeks later that Dr. Khabbaz had text messaged my cardiologist, Dr. Kalin, at 11:00 p.m. that night to tell him the surgery went well. These guys worked long hours.

The remainder of the day was a blur. At some stage they took the oxygen mask off my mouth and nose, replacing it with two plastic tubes in my nostrils. About every four hours they came by to check my vitals: blood pressure, oxygen intake, weight, and heart rate.

There were wire electrodes that entered my body about four inches above my groin, and they sent messages to a monitor screen at the nurse's station and a monitor screen in my room. The screen showed a continuous graph of heart rhythm, blood pressure, oxygen intake, and heartbeat.

I think many people are worried before open-heart surgery (OHS), specifically about whether they will suffer pain. While lying down during surgery and in the ICU you can feel pain in the muscles in your chest, shoulders, and back, but all this is taken care of with painkillers. They ask you every four hours if you have pain and on a scale from zero to ten.

They gave me two painkillers every four hours, if I needed it. I went through the whole time in hospital with virtually no pain.

The next day was the day before Thanksgiving. I had an appetite, which I was told was a good sign. They gave me a little scrambled eggs and toast and coffee for breakfast.

Adele arrived at 1:00 p.m. She had gone back to the Cape, picked up Bella from our friends, and returned with Bella and booked into the hotel opposite the hospital. My dear wife came back again at 3:00 and again at 7:00, each time returning to the hotel to find Bella on the bed watching Animal Planet.

I don't remember much of the first day in the ICU, except for the continual *beep, beep, beep* from heart monitors. They'd alert the staff if someone stopped breathing.

I remember saying to one of the nurses my arm was aching, and then a little later I said my back side was aching. She replied in a jesting manner, "I know you are just one big ache." It made me laugh, and she gave me a shot of something, probably morphine, in both places. That took care of that. Aching occurs because the body is in one position for hours at a time.

That night Kevin and Mike were the nurses on duty. I vaguely remember being bathed in bed. This was the first time after the surgery. Apparently Kevin lived in Maine and traveled down three times a week. He kindly told me he comforted Adele when she rang at 10:00 p.m.

That night they removed the catheter from my body. That was good news because it was a sure sign of moving forward. It also meant I could get out of bed more easily and go the bathroom on my own.

The next day was Thanksgiving. A pleasant smiling face appeared over my bed and presented me with oatmeal, scrambled eggs, toast, and coffee on a tray for breakfast.

Adele arrived around 9:00 a.m. and stayed for an hour. I said I felt like resting, and I wanted her to go to her brother Ronnie's home, where they were hosting Thanksgiving. All her family would be there.

Donna and Carol were the nurses on duty. Donna mentioned that all the nurses and staff had brought in some food, and they were all going to pool it and celebrate Thanksgiving when they could, in the breaks they got. She also mentioned the hospital was putting on a Thanksgiving turkey dinner in the restaurant for all the staff at 7:00 p.m. She said, "I'll be too full to go to that!"

I was told later that Dr. Allison was to change the large tube in the left side of my neck to a smaller one. The smaller one was left in the neck right up until I left the hospital. It served as an entry for medication if my condition took a turn for the worse.

I was half asleep but heard Donna and Carol talking. I looked up and saw a steel railing above me. "Heck! What is this?"

"You are a bit of a worrier," Carol said. "It is a hoist so we can lift you higher into the bed."

After that was achieved, Dr. Allison arrived to change the tube in my neck. "Turn your head to the left." The good doctor then proceeded to work on my neck. It felt like someone nibbling and poking about at the same spot for about fifteen, minutes: *peck, peck,* ouch, *peck,* aah, aah.

I said, "It feels like Dracula is working on my neck!" As soon as I had said it, I thought that didn't sound right. She might take revenge. So I said, "An attractive Dracula."

"Oh that's nice," she said dryly.

I heard them discussing whether they should give me one or two Percocet for the pain. Someone said, "Two."

Sometime later I heard two people talking from about a million miles away. I stirred and said, "I am off the planet."

"You're a cheap date," one of the nurses said.

I had never taken these painkillers before, and fortunately I was able to drop off them about a week after I left the hospital. However, I knew this whole procedure would've been a nightmare without them—probably impossible.

Adele returned again about 6:30 p.m., stayed an hour, and then went back to the hotel.

Donna told me our good friends from New Hampshire, Charlie and Allison, had wanted to send flowers.

Unfortunately they didn't accept flowers in the ICU. I guess they didn't want any bugs crawling around in there.

That evening my mother-in-law, Roxy, and my brother-in-law Ronnie, were coming to see me on Thanksgiving evening. I told Adele that I was not feeling up to seeing visitors yet; I felt tired and needed to rest, but I said that I would see them soon. I greatly appreciated their love and support, but I just didn't feel up to visitors, even family.

The same applied the next day, when my brother-in-law Anan, my sister-in-law Stephanie, and their daughter and my goddaughter Anjali were coming to see me.

I said, "Save the trip, and I'll see you soon." My family gave great encouragement and support at this time, and I was very thankful for it. One of the great things about times like these is having the support of family and friends.

They were going to keep me another night in the ICU, but I asked if I could be moved out and onto the floor below. The activity in ICU was incredible. Doctors came and went, and there was the continual noise of mechanical beeps, buzzes, and patients! Thankfully there was a room available in the Farr Building on the sixth floor, which was another part of the center. They put me in a wheelchair and gave me a ride to the room.

The nurses, doctors and staff I came in contact with everywhere were friendly and showed they wanted to help. Lucy arrived with her happy yellow bow in her hair and gleaming white teeth. "Here is your dinner, Roger: baked cod, mash, corn, apple juice, and coffee." Kate and Christen were the nurses on duty that evening. Christen was going to see her family on Long Island the next day, and Kate mentioned she had been through the same surgery I had had, so she knew what I was going through.

I slept like a log that night.

The next day was Black Friday. Lucy arrived and placed a tray over my bed: scrambled eggs, toast, apple juice, and coffee for breakfast.

They give you a little red pillow in the shape of a heart. It becomes your best friend. You hug it against your chest whenever you get out of bed, or whenever you have the urge to cough. It took the pressure of your chest and helped the movement to be less painful. You use it all the way up to about two weeks after arriving home. They also give you a plastic devise that is called an incentive spirometer. It is a hard plastic cylinder with a rubber tube attached, which you put in your mouth and suck air out of, and you are asked to use it every hour or so. You must empty your lungs and suck as much air as you can, then hold your breath for as long as possible. There is a red marker that indicates what figure you achieved. You are forever trying to beat the figure you achieved the time before. It is a very important tool because it keeps your lungs dry and can prevent you from catching pneumonia.

As soon as I mastered the art of getting out of bed by hugging the little red pillow, rolling my shoulder to the side of the bed, and easing my feet out of the bed, I started an exercise that gave me quick progress. Normally you have to wait for the physiotherapist to come by and help you go for a walk down the corridor. When they do that, they put a safety belt around your waist, which they hold in case you start to fall. They will not let you leave the hospital until you can walk down three corridors and walk up two flights of stairs, so there is real incentive to get on with it. My method was to ease myself out of bed, sit on the edge of the bed for a few minutes with the pillow held tightly against me, say "One, two, three," and then pull myself to standing position. I would grab hold of the edge of the table they have to swing over my bed and start marching on the spot. I did this regularly and sometimes at night while I watched television. It gave me my strength in quicker than normal time. In fact one of the nurses was surprised I had made it to the bathroom in my room by myself ahead of schedule. After surgery they basically had to help me start walking again.

At around 11:00 a.m. Audra was showing me how to bathe my new zipper. "You have to use Ivory soap and not any scented soaps. Wash every day and pat dry with a soft towel."

Suddenly Adele arrived with Bella, our golden retriever. She is a companion dog and was allowed in hospitals. Adele wanted to bring her into the ICU, and the nurses said she would be allowed. I didn't want Bella coming to the ICU; it wasn't necessary, and I felt uncomfortable about it.

Adele looked a little taken aback when she saw the incision, which stretched fourteen inches from my neck to my stomach. Nowadays they do not stitch it up anymore—they glue it up, believe it or not. Later when I was bathing the scar, I could see the clear, rubberlike substance that eventually melts away. The incision finishes up looking like a fine line rather than a zipper.

Adele and Bella left after an hour or so, booked out of the hotel, and drove back to the Cape. I had been given the clearance to be able to leave the hospital the next day, which was a Saturday.

It was amazing: I had surgery on my heart on Tuesday, and I was going home on Saturday, four days later. I couldn't believe it.

The plan was Adele would drive back the next day without Bella and pick me up. I had to sit in the back seat of the car to avoid getting hit in the chest by an air bag, in the unfortunate case of an accident.

That afternoon the doctor came by to remove the wire electrodes in my body that led directly to the heart. Taking out these wires was definitely not great fun.

Dr. Jennifer sailed into the room with a mission, full of good humor. "Hi, Mr. Kohler. Do you mind if I call you Roger?"

"No, not at all."

"I have to remove the box above your groin, with the wires going into your heart."

"Oh, that sounds fun!" I said sarcastically.

"It will hurt a little, but I will tell you when to hold your breath."

"Man, that sounds a bit of a worry."

She played around there at the spot about four inches north-northeast of my belly button for about two minutes. "Hold your breath."

I sucked in some air. "Whoooooof … Yikes!"

"All done!"

After that, I could imagine anyone who saw her coming down the pike and knew her job would run at a hundred miles per hour in the opposite direction.

I picked up the phone and rang in an order for dinner: salmon, potatoes, canned peaches, apple juice, and coffee.

A Song from Heaven

It was Saturday morning, and I was going home in the afternoon. The sun was beaming in through the window, and I was already feeling better than before the surgery. I ordered oatmeal, toast and jelly, orange juice, and coffee for breakfast.

The nurse came by and said, "The doctor will be coming by to pull the other wire electrodes from your heart, near where the others were."

"Oh, I didn't know there were any others." I remembered the last time experience with wire pulling. It was the only time I'd felt a little pain since being in the hospital.

Dr. Jennifer wasn't around today, so Dr. Sue was to do the task. She sailed into my room and told me that unfortunately she would not be able to pull the wires because my blood thickness was 2.4 INR and it had to be 2.0 INR or lower to avoid bleeding. The higher the number, the bigger the chance the blood wouldn't coagulate if I bled. They gave me medication to lower the figure.

The bad news was that I would be going home tomorrow, and not today. I had to phone Adele and give her the news. She replied, "Oh, well that is disappointing, but better to be sure and not sorry."

On two occasions I had a young nurse come to take an X-ray while I was in bed. These nurses must be in their early twenties, and they have very good bedside manner. They wheel in a machine, pulled me up off the pillow, and placed a hard metal sheet against my back. Then they jammed the front of the machine against my chest while breathing clean, sweet breath all over me, like a breath of fresh air. They then withdrew behind a screen and told me to hold my breath. I heard a buzz, and then they said, "Okay, we are done." They withdrew the sheet from behind me and were gone.

It was Saturday night, and Adam and Sean came at 7:00. I had baked cod, potatoes, corn, apple juice, and coffee for dinner.

I was due for another bathing. Being washed in bed by two males was a new one for me, and it was the second time in a week. I said to Sean, "So I suppose at 7:00 a.m. when you leave here, you go and have a big breakfast at some great diner around here?"

"No, I go home, walk the dog, and fall into bed."

These nurses worked twelve-hour shifts, from seven to seven, and they did it three or four times a week.

Adam said to me, "Where is that accent from?"

"Australia," I replied. "I'll bet yours is from Switzerland."

"No, Poland."

"Oh, really? I love Addinsell's *Warsaw Concerto*."

He didn't answer. I guess he didn't hear me, or he didn't like it.

Adam rides a bicycle to work. He must get up at 4:00 a.m. and ride to the hospital in near freezing temperatures in winter. Now there is a good American.

I said to Mike, "Where is your accent from?"

"Boston."

"Oh, sorry. I thought you sounded a bit Irish."

He laughed. "No, I'm a Bostonian."

Sean looked like a body builder. I asked if he could help me get out of bed to go to the bathroom.

He picked me up, all two hundred pounds, like a feather and stood me up.

Later that night the phone rang. "Hey, Roger, it's Charlie. How are you doing?"

"Hi, Charlie. I'm doing great."

I was not in the mood for a long conversation, but great to hear from a good friend.

Patients are encouraged to walk about if they can, to improve their condition and speed recovery. I grabbed my little red pillow, made it out of bed, and with slow paces wobbled down the corridor. I took a left at the nurse's station and headed down to the sitting area at the end of the hall. The room has floor-to-ceiling windows, and because it's on the sixth floor, it looks out over a park in Brookline. It was 3:00 a.m. *The Wizard of Oz* was on television, on low volume. I sat for ten minutes and then headed back to the room. There was a large red box, in the shape of a heart, of Stover chocolates on the counter at the nurse's station. I was tempted to indulge but refrained.

It was now Sunday morning, and I was going home in the afternoon. Dr. Allison arrived to pull the wires. My blood was now 2.0 LNR, so she could do the job.

Dr. Jennifer had used the "Hold your breath, fast pull" method. Dr. Allison was going to use the "Hold your breath slowly, slowly catchy monkey" method. She played around there at a spot about four inches north-northwest of my belly button for about two minutes. "Hold your breath. How is the property market at the moment?"

You know how your dentist is always asking you questions when there are about four steel things hanging out of your mouth? Or you are in a restaurant, and the waitress asks, "How is everything so far?" when you have your mouth full of food?

"Ahh … Yikes!"

"All done," she said.

"Ma'am, thank goodness that's over."

A few moments after the wires were pulled, I started feeling these erratic explosions in my heart. They were so strong, or at least felt that way, that I could see the sheets covering my chest bouncing up and down. Then it stopped.

A moment later the doctor appeared at the door of the room. She had obviously seen what had happened on the screen at the nurse's station. "Are you all right?"

"I think so. Man, that was scary."

The doctor said that it was the heart settling down after the change. I'd had a feeling of anxiety. "I think we should keep you here another night."

I said, "Okay, that sounds good to me." It gave me a fright and I didn't want that sort of fright happening at home.

When I knew I was staying another night, my heart beat and vital readings returned to normal, or so I was told.

I started feeling really good after a while and then decided to phone Adele and tell her what had happened.

She was disappointed that I would be delayed another day, but she agreed that it was the smartest thing to do.

It felt like my heart was a little person inside me that said, "I didn't like what you just did," and then it started punching me.

I was lying there, and I could hear a soft singing coming down the hallway. The singing gradually got louder, and then in came the happy, smiling face of a lady with beautiful teeth.

I said, "Hi, you have a beautiful voice. What were you singing?"

"Oh, some music from the church."

"Gosh, it was so soothing. What is your name?"

She replied, "Susanna—you know, like in the song." She spoke with a very Southern accent.

"Can you sing me a song?" I asked.

"Sure, what do you want me to sing?"

"Oh, whatever you would like to sing."

"Sure, only I can't sing in English."

I said, "That's fine. What would you like to sing it in?"

"Creole," she said. "I'm from Haiti."

"That would be marvelous."

She stood at the doorway of the room, holding a broom at forty-five degrees, her head held high, her eyes looking toward the heavens. Then she broke forth with a beautiful song. The room filled with sunlight. It felt as though there may have been an angel somewhere in the room.

When she had finished she looked back at me with a beautiful, big smile on her face.

"That was marvelous," I said, clapping. "Maybe you can come by again tomorrow and sing me another."

"Sure!" And with that, she moved off down the hallway, swishing her broom and singing softly.

In the other section of the room was Mr. Wang, a friendly, smiling gentleman from Taiwan. He spoke broken English, and I guess had a lady come by to help him order meals at mealtime.

I gather this was a service of the hospital, if one wanted it. The other method was to consult a menu on your table and place an order of what you wanted with the kitchen on the phone. This is the method I used.

Lucy would come by around at 7:00 a.m., 11:00 a.m., and 4:00 p.m. to take Mr. Wang's order. She always wore yellow, which looked so happy against the other colors in the hospital, and she wore a big yellow bow in her hair.

"Hello, Mr. Wang, what you like today?"

I have to say the food was good. On the second night in the hospital, I remember saying to the lady who took the trays back to the kitchen, "My compliments to the chef."

The nurse in the room said, "Are you serious?"

I said, "Yes, absolutely." Maybe after you have had your chest opened up, all food tastes good.

No, joking aside, I thought the food was good, though not the Ritz, mind you.

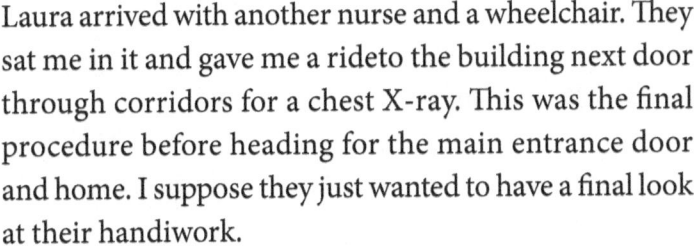

Laura arrived with another nurse and a wheelchair. They sat me in it and gave me a ride to the building next door through corridors for a chest X-ray. This was the final procedure before heading for the main entrance door and home. I suppose they just wanted to have a final look at their handiwork.

I was certainly ready and thinking of going home the next day after being delayed twice before, once because my blood was to thin to pull the wires the first time, and then the second time because of the palpitations in my heart after the wires were pulled. Still, I was amazed I was going home six days after open-heart surgery.

Suddenly I had a dreadful thought. *Holy mackerel, I have a big problem.* I pressed the button for the nurse.

A voice from a speaker on the wall above my bed, which was connected to the nurse's center said, "Yes, Mr. Kohler, can we help you?"

"Yes, I need to talk to the nurse."

The day duty nurse came into the room.

"Laura, I hate to surprise you, but I have a big problem."

"Really? What is it?"

"You know I am supposed to go home tomorrow afternoon?"

"Yes ..."

"I am sorry to tell you this, but it has just dawned on me that I remember being told that a patient cannot leave without them having had a proper bowel movement with soft stool."

"Yes."

"Well, I have had about fifteen bowel movements, but when I think about it, it was always gas."

She said, "When you told us you were having bowel movements, someone should have been looking to see what passes. Have they?"

"I am not sure."

"Okay, no problem. We will sort this out by the time I finish today."

"Really, what time is that?"

"At 7:30 p.m. I will be back with prune juice."

In came two glasses of prune juice. Down the hatch they went.

Laura returned a short time later with a capsule of stool softener. Down the hatch.

About twenty minutes later, Laura was back with milk of magnesia. This was a white substance with very little taste, and it was taken with a full glass of water. Down the hatch.

By the time two hours had passed, there was no action.

Laura said, "This will eventually happen."

I replied, "I hope so—I am beginning to feel pregnant. Laura, I want to be out of here tomorrow. I am feeling okay, and I really have to get home if I can, because my wife has been coming here from the Cape, and it is a two-hour ride each way".

"Okay, we will try from both ends."

Next came a suppository, which was a white horse pill of gel that was inserted with gel.

"Oh, Oh!"

One hour later, still nothing.

I got out of bed, walked down to the nurse's station, and said to Laura, "If I have three or four more glasses of prune juice, this has got to happen, surely?"

"Yes, probably, but first I am going to try an enema as well. I think that should do it."

"Oh, really?"

I went back to bed feeling exhausted. I fell half asleep, and Laura returned twenty minutes later with the equipment.

I said, "I'm half asleep."

She said, "Don't worry—this will soon wake you up."

A plastic tube was inserted, and a cool, soft gel was slowly injected. "Ooohhh ..."

Laura was due to leave at 7:30 p.m. At 7:25 she returned and said, "I'm sure this will do the trick." She put two glasses of warm prune juice on my table.

Down the hatch.

I said, "I feel it is going to happen, and soon."

At 8:00 sharp, I made the ten-second dash to the bathroom. Man, was that a load off my mind. Now I could go home tomorrow.

That Sunday night I watched Fox. There was a program on about the coming of the end of the world, according to predications from the Mayan times. "Good Grief, I have just had heart surgery that may extend my life for another twenty or thirty years, and the world is going to end in four weeks? Fortunately they were saying most experts discounted the theory.

In the rooms they had small plastic bags of antiseptic wipes. They were small sheets of tissues, wet and cool, to be used for wiping your hands, but they advised patients not to use them on the face. They are on the side table and on the tray table.

I had noticed I had developed an itching rash on my back, probably from sweating a bit and being on my back for five days. I used these wipes on my back. The sensation was amazing, cool, and slightly stinging. The relief was like heaven, and the rash was gone in twenty-four hours.

Recovery

The next morning Audra and Donna were on duty. Lucy arrived smiling as always, with my breakfast: oatmeal, toast, and coffee. Mr. Wang was up, sitting in a chair and looking out the window. It was one of those beautiful Boston mornings, cool with a deep blue sky.

Audra came in to remove the bandage on my incision and any other bandages I had on my arms where tubes were attached. We got talking about dogs, and out came her smart phone to show me her pit bull and pretty daughter. She provided me with all those things needed for a shower and toiletry.

Audra had warned me about giving me a fine if I didn't brush my teeth, so I said, "Can you please give me another tooth brush? I don't want to get a fine."

I had my first shower since surgery, and it was really something, probably the best shower of my life.

"You are going home today, right?" Audra asked.

"Yes, ma'am."

"Don't go back to work for a few weeks."

"I won't."

"Good, I live in Andover, and I'll be looking out for you."

"Oh, Okay. That means if I come into the Andover area, I'd better be wearing my Gaucho Marx mustache," I joked. "No, I won't be going back to work for a while. I would hate to undo all the good work you nurses do."

I was given the okay to dress, and Donna came to instruct me about the medications I was to take, nine in all. It was the hospitals responsibility to explain what the medications were for.

- Amiodarone 400mg, then 200mg after one week, and discontinue after one month (for heart rhythm)
- Baby aspirin, 90mg
- Docusate sodium, 200mg (stool softener)
- Furosemide, 40mg (for water removal)
- Lisinopril, 10mg (for blood pressure)

- Metoprolol, 25mg. (for blood pressure)
- Oxycodone, 5–325mg (painkiller)
- Potassium chloride (for water loss)
- Coumiden, 1–5mg (blood thinner)

Donna then presented me with all the paperwork for hospital release. She had me sign the hospital release, and then came the important instructions about what not to do at home.

- No lifting anything over ten pounds for ten weeks.
- No snow shoveling
- No vacuuming
- No driving for four weeks
- Ride in the back seat going home, to avoid air bags.
- Get plenty of rest
- Rest after exercise
- Rest after showering
- Rest after eating
- Don't walk your dog on a leash

I had read in the literature for taking Coumiden that I had to take great care not to cut myself, especially when using sharp objects like knives, scissors, and garden tools. Coumiden is a blood-thinning drug, and bleeding is harder to stop because the blood does not coagulate as easily. It is recommended to use an electric shaver. Adele, being observant, had gone out and bought me the latest Braun shaver. The last one I had was about forty years ago.

I had been told I could leave the hospital around 12:30 p.m. I had already informed Adele at 10:00 a.m. because she had a two-hour ride from the Cape. Adele, who was adored by every dog she met, arrived at noon and heard the medications described, and then all three of us went to the main entrance of the hospital.

Donna said good-bye, Adele went to get the car, and we headed back to the Cape. I was in a very talkative mood; I think the narcotic painkillers made everyone that way.

When we arrived home, I went into the living room, switched on the television, and sat down on the sofa. "Honey, did you buy a new television?" I asked.

"No."

Before the surgery, the television was very blurred, and I was contemplating buying glasses to view it. Now it was crystal clear. I couldn't believe it! I guess having a more efficient heart improved my vision.

We decided to take a photo of the incision. We then looked at the last photo of me before the surgery, and sure enough, I looked far better now, with the other photo showing me with a puffy face.

About two hours after we arrived home, Rachael, the case manager from Visiting Nurses Association of Cape Cod, arrived. She was immaculately dressed in her little white outfit, looking like the perfect nurse out of a storybook.

"I need to take your blood sample to check the INR." She produced a gadget to prick my fingered, and she put the drop of blood onto the little machine. She said the reading was 3.2 and in the correct range. My blood had to be between 2.5 INR and 3.5 INR.

A nurse called a little later to tell me how much Coumiden (blood thinner) to take for the next three days.

Rachael then checked I had been given an exercise program at the hospital, and she asked whether I would need a physical therapist to come to our home. I said I had a program from the hospital, and I wouldn't need a physio. She asked if I had all the info about my medications. I said yes. Last she wanted to know that I was fully informed about diet during recovery.

With that, she departed in her little white car. I was very impressed.

A nurse—Beverly, Judy, Becky, or Carol—came every three or four days to check my INR reading for the next four weeks. They continued this until I was able to go the local C-Lab once a month to have my INR checked.

Ellen and Holly often called on the telephone from the VNA office, to chat about the readings from the little black box.

Ellen called on a regular basis for weeks, until I was driving and no longer needed the VNA. She was always so interested in my progress, and it was a very comforting feeling.

It was on the third day home that Cathy from VNA had arrived with the little black box. The box was plugged into a power and telephone outlet. It recorded and sent to their office my vitals every day until they decided I had fully recovered from the open-heart surgery. This was taking good care of me even while I was at home.

The time is set on the machine; in my case it's 7:00 a.m.

I'm lying in bed and then hear, "Good morning, it is time to check your vitals. Please step on the scales."

"Please step off the scales."

"Please sit down in front of the machine. Please put the blood pressure cuff on your right arm just above the elbow and tighten it."

"Please put the finger sensor on your middle finger on your left arm. Please rest your arm as instructed by the clinician."

"Please press the green start button."

Buzz. The arm sleeve tightens and then loosens.

The machine asks you questions. "Please press the yes or no buttons following these questions."

"Are you experiencing difficulty breathing?"

"Are you experiencing any dizziness?"

"Are your ankles swollen?"

"Thank you. Please remember to take your medications and eat a proper diet."

Then four readings (blood pressure, heart rate, oxygen intake, and weight) appear on the front of the box, and they are transmitted to the VNA office.

If any of the readings were not as they should have been, then Ellen or Holly would phone to see how I was.

Often, I would receive a call from Ellen or Holly. "Hi, Roger, how are you doing today?"

Very impressive. I always felt they were taking good care of me.

In this way I am at home, and they are watching my condition all the way until I am completely recovered.

I started with nine medications to take when I left the hospital. After ten days I was down to six. The painkillers were needed less frequently, and I was off the potassium and off the lasic (water pill). I was continuing with two pills for blood pressure, one for heart rhythm, one for stool softener, and the Coumiden (blood thinner).

After ten days I received a call from Dr. Kalin's office asking me to increase my dose of the blood pressure pills.

It became a fairly simple plan each day of exercise, watch my diet, take my medications, and rest.

When you take the medication Coumiden (blood thinner), you are given plenty of literature about it, and you have to watch your diet because there are certain foods you have to avoid. You are required to avoid foods containing vitamin K. That suited me. Brussels sprouts, spinach, broccoli, dark green lettuce—these were never on my favorites list.

In the following days I started to feel my heart was operating far more efficiently. It felt like it was operating at 100 percent, whereas before the surgery it felt it was operating at about 60 percent.

The painkiller given to me at the hospital—which believe me is essential—is called Percocet, pronounced "Perk-o-set." This is funny because when I asked Adele if my painkiller made me any different to how I was normally, she said, "It makes you more perky!" When these ran out after a week at home, I was perfectly happy to go onto Hydrocoden, which is a painkiller but a step down from the narcotic Percocet, whose prescription cannot be faxed to pharmacies. It can be prescribed but has to be handed directly to you. That would have been a problem for me because it meant a four-hour round trip to Boston.

The Hydrocoden worked fine with me the first time I used it. I continued to need painkillers occasionally for another two weeks.

Our good friends from New Hampshire, Ellen and Keith, sent me a box from Edible Arrangements: chocolate covered strawberries. This was one of the advantages of being a patient.

After two weeks at home and twenty days after the surgery, I was feeling so well and recovering quickly that I was thinking about the shortness of time. Thinking about time reminded me of a story an attorney told me years ago. An attorney asked a judge, "When do you think you will make your deliberations?"

The judge replied, "All in the goodness of time." That could mean three days, three weeks, or three years.

I had always been a little worried about the noise I had been told the mechanical valve made. Now three weeks after the surgery, I knew all of the doctors who had said, "It is not a problem," were right. Someone had said it was a clicking noise. I would describe it as a ticking noise. It reminded me of the fine tick, tick, of a Rolex watch. I could hear it sometimes, but as soon as I turned my mind to any thought at all, it disappeared.

Before the surgery I had felt tired and thought, *Oh, I'm just getting old. Probably not eating the right diet, not exercising enough.* No, it was a problem with my heart! I needed a new valve in my heart because the original one had worn out.

There must be thousands of folks out there who are feeling tired and think, *Oh, I'm just getting old.* Then they go about their daily lives as I was, having never had any chest pains, dizziness, numbness, or any other apparent heart attack signs and are heading for a heart attack and they don't know it.

After having my surgery and feeling the huge difference with the new valve, I feel sure I would have had a heart attack in short time if I hadn't had the surgery.

After I had been home for three weeks, I called a friend and neighbor, Harry, to give him the heads–up on my recovery. I could not believe what he told me. A close friend of his had suffered a heart attack, falling over in his living room with his seven-year-old granddaughter being the only one home. The small girl called 911, and when they arrived, the man was dead. Here is someone who obviously had a heart problem and didn't know it.

A Remarkable Experience

You might well wonder what one might do while being homebound for weeks on end before being able to leave the house and drive again. I found reading a great pastime. One of my favorite authors is Paul Theroux. Funnily enough, he lives on Cape Cod at East Sandwich for six months of the year; the other six he lives in Hawaii. I have ten of his travel books, and they sit on my bedside table. The great thing about these books is that you can pick up any one of them and open it up anywhere, and start reading. You may be rattling along in a train in Sri Lanka heading to Colombo from Galle along the coast, with the sea spray hitting the windows. Or you could be climbing a mountain in a train in Burma past beautiful scenery heading for Mandalay to visit Mr. Bernard. Or you could be traveling with Duffill, who he later thought was a spy, on the Direct Orient Express from Paris to Istanbul. Or you'll be sitting on a train stopped in the middle of a high, grassy field in India, where he could only imagine the train driver had hopped off the train to relieve himself. Then you pick up another one and open it somewhere, and you read about him sleeping on a bench on a lonely, dust-blown railway station at 3:00 a.m. in Patagonia.

It also gave me timeto catch up with family members by e-mail: my daughter in Singapore, my sons in Australia, and my cousin in Zurich, Switzerland.

Of course, another good pastime was sitting snoozing in a recliner and listening to Beethoven's *Fourth Symphony*.

I found myself listening to a set of eight CDs called "The Classic 100 ". It is a collection of one hundred classical music masterpieces compiled by the ABC (Australian Broadcasting Corporation) a few years ago. They asked their listeners to submit their favorite piece of classical music (a piece of music they couldn't live without) and then compiled the one hundred most favorite pieces on eight CDs. This collection plays for a little more than ten hours. The list starts with Mozart and finishes with Faure. Composers include Mozart, Vaughan Williams, Beethoven, Bizet, Handel, Strauss, Bach, Rachmaninov, Bruch, Vivaldi, Schubert, Elgar, Puccini, Verdi, Massenet, Mahler, Saint-Saens, Gluck, Wagner, Dvorak, Prokofiev, Elgar, Smetana, Tchaikovsky, Grieg, Chopin, Gershwin, Ravel, Mendelssohn, Sibelius, Purcell, Debussy, Albinoni,

Stravinsky, Khachaturian and Faure. Included in the collection is George Gershwin's "Rhapsody in Blue", with George Gershwin playing the piano, recorded on 10 June 1924 in New York.

It is fantastic listening because it is such a wide variety of classical music.

I regularly listened to the Cape Cod classical station 107.5 and it is good but they do give Haydn a bit of a hidin'.

We moved to New England years ago to be close to Adele's dad, who was having failing health and lived in Andover, Massachusetts. Sadly Ed passed away three years ago. He was the nicest man I'd ever met. A recent Mike Huckabee program mentioned 1 Samuel 16:7, "Man looks at the outward appearance, but the Lord Looks at the Heart." This reminded me of Ed.

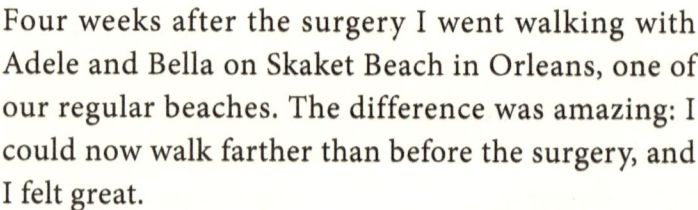

Four weeks after the surgery I went walking with Adele and Bella on Skaket Beach in Orleans, one of our regular beaches. The difference was amazing: I could now walk farther than before the surgery, and I felt great.

After four weeks I was allowed to drive again, so I started to head back to the office. I got a great reception there, with everyone seemingly surprised that I was out and about so soon. I think I was surprised as well.

I headed down to Larry's in Chatham for a little lunch. Debbie was there and came to ask what I would like for lunch. She said I looked great and asked how it all went. I responded, "Great!"

Larry's is one of those seaside diners where customers get a hearty meal at a reasonable price. I remember when I went there first a few years ago, and an elderly gentleman, probably around eighty, was straightening out menus and collecting plates from tables. He walked past me at the bar and was a little bent over, moving slowly. I said, "You must be Larry."

He replied in a softly spoken voice, "No, I'm Larry's son."

Gosh, I thought, *Larry must be in the kitchen and is probably 103.* You can always tell when you go there if the Boston Red Sox won or lost, by Debbie's mood.

My wife had mentioned many times about a rehabilitation center at Falmouth, where patients are invited to attend to help with getting back on track physically and mentally, with education classes provided. As I was now driving, I thought I would go and check it out.

I phoned the Cardiac Rehabilitation Center at Falmouth Hospital and spoke to Sheri. She gave me the hours and told me about the program. Then she said, "Please come and join us."

I drove to the center and was welcomed. There were lots of smiling faces of people, with more women than I was expecting. Patients were pedaling bicycles, rowing machines, walking on treadmills, and pushing weights.

The mood was happy and enthusiastic. I guessed they were people who were happy to be given another chance of living longer.

The staff there were always friendly. They got great satisfaction from this job because they found it so rewarding.

The manager Susan Crider, RN does a great job and makes you feel welcome.

This center had comprehensive exercises and educational program designed to help the individual to make the lifestyle changes needed to improve cardiovascular health. There were thirty-six sessions that go for twelve weeks. The group exercise sessions met on Mondays, Wednesdays, and Fridays. Sessions consisted of exercise using stationary bikes, treadmills, rowing machines, arm exercises, and hand weights. EKG machines were provided to monitor progress, and it was supervised by exercise specialists and experienced cardiac nurses. They said that 95 percent of people who attended said it improved their lifestyle in regard to cardiovascular health.

I decided to attend the center for a month or so. Why not see what they have to say? It also gave one a great chance to meet other people in the same predicament, and hear their stories.

After the exercise class, a class of information followed, where a supervisor told us about changing our lifestyle to help with a longer life.

Since the surgery I had been eating far less. The problem was that many restaurants loaded plates up with huge servings, and for me it caused a problem because I came from a modest family upbringing, where my mother told us we must eat everything on our plates.

I had discovered—and I wish I had years earlier—that the best idea was to remove half the food on the plate to a side dish, to take home.

I slowly started to return to the office again on a regular basis. I was totally surprised to find our office was being renovated. I had a renovated heart, and I was now getting a renovated office to boot! They were doing a spectacular job. New hardwood floors, new blue carpet with white stars, new lighting, new desks, new everything. It was a great job. A few people were saying, "It will be great when it is finished."

My tough-minded father would have summed the renovation up by saying, "They do a lot in a long time."

My father always suffered from sea sickness throughout his life; in fact he often joked that he got sea sick when he stood on a dock.

Occasionally I went for a quick breakfast at the Hole In One in Orleans, another one of those great eateries on the Cape. At 8:00 a.m. on a Friday and Saturday in the summer, there are twenty people sitting around outside waiting for table. Funnily enough, a Debbie also works there. She is a great source of information about Caribbean cruises. She was telling me one day about a cruise one could get on out of Florida for twenty-five dollars a day.

Pretty amazing. If you keep an eye on these cruise ships, they offer incredible last-minute deals to fill cabins. It is surprising what you can learn from restaurants.

Lori, the owner of the restaurant, said, "Hi, Roger. We haven't seen you for a while. We guessed you were on vacation."

I replied, "Yes I have been … at the Beth Israel Five Star in Boston, and it was all good."

All's Well that Ends Well

Heart valve disease occurs when a valve doesn't work right. A valve may not open all the way, or a valve may have problems closing. If this occurs, blood doesn't move through the heart's chambers the way it should.

If a valve does open all the way, the blood moves through to the next chamber. If a valve doesn't close tightly, blood can leak backward. This problem means the heart must work harder to pump the same amount of blood, or blood may back up in the lungs or body because it is not running through the heart as it should.

Regurgitation results when the valve doesn't close tightly, and the blood leaks back the wrong way through the valve. In other words, the blood is not going to the aorta and on to the body, but back into the heart. This is the problem I had.

Aortic stenosis is when the aortic valve becomes too narrow and in turn reduces the amount of blood that can flow through it. If the narrowing is mild, the overall performance of the heart may not be reduced. However, the valve can become so narrow (stenotic) that the heart function is reduced, and the rest of the body may not receive adequate blood flow.

Initial symptoms of aortic valve disease or regurgitation are:

- fatigue
- easy tiring
- loss of energy
- swelling of the ankles
- palpitations (extra or skipped heartbeat)

More advanced symptoms are:

- shortness of breath
- chest pains
- dizziness or loss of consciousness

The symptoms I was experiencing were tiredness and fatigue, and I really didn't know these were dangerous signs; I thought it was pretty normal for someone who was sixty-six years old.

The danger is thinking this, because you can be ***heading for a heart attack and not know it.***

The other sign is when a doctor tells you have a heart murmur. A heart murmur represents turbulent blood flow across an abnormal valve—a sign you could need valve replacement or surgery. I have had people tell me they have had a heart murmur for years. I think those people need to have an echocardiogram done, and soon.

The ***echocardiogram takes only forty minutes*** and is a specialized heart ultrasound which allows the doctor to visualize and listen to the heart valve and determine the severity and possible cause of aortic valve disease.

A study from the University of Southern California Keck School of Medicine shows coronary artery disease is a leading health problem in the United States.

According to the most recent figures from the American Heart Association, ***coronary heart disease is the single leading cause of death in America today.***

More than twelve million people alive today have a history of heart attack, angina pectoris (chest pain), or both. ***An estimated 1.1 million Americans will have a new or recurrent coronary attack this year—and one-third of the patients will die.***

Coronary artery disease patients are usually men over the age of sixty-five. Historically, coronary artery disease has been considered a men's disease, but it is also *the largest cause of death among women in the United States.* According to the National Institute of Health, African American women in particular are 24 percent more likely to die of coronary artery disease than their Caucasian American counterparts. Older women also have significantly higher possibility of coronary artery disease than younger women. On average, women develop coronary artery disease fifteen years later than men, but 39 percent of women die from the disease as compared to 31 percent of men.

The surgery team for heart valve surgery includes:

- surgeon
- assistant surgeon
- cardiologist
- surgical nurse
- perfusionist
- anesthesiologist
- nurse

The anesthesiologist constantly monitors your anesthesia to help you sleep without pain. Your blood pressure, temperature, and breathing are constantly monitored on a screen during surgery.

The perfusionist operates the heart-lung bypass machine, which keeps your blood flowing during the surgery. When they are operating on your heart, they actually stop your heart beating when they stitch in a new valve, and then they restart the beating. The warmth of the blood restarts your heart when they turn off the heart-lung bypass machine. If your heart does not restart, then they give you medication, sometimes more than once.

Joel Osteen mentioned on his much-watched Sunday service broadcast on several TV channels that seven million people watch, in one hundred nations around the world, with his congregation of forty thousand, that he knew a women who had heart bypass surgery. When the warmth of the blood and the medication didn't work, the surgeon started gently massaging her heart, leaned over the top of the patient, and said, "Mary, I need you to restart your heart."

Immediately her heart started to beat again. I hope a few surgeons read this book, although they probably know that story already.

I think Joel does an outstanding job in giving people tremendous encouragement in his weekly broadcast and service in the Lakewood Church in Houston, Texas, and I truly believe that with the help of God, he saves lives.

If you want a good laugh on a Sunday morning, watch Joel on the Discovery Channel. As he delivers his message of hope and encouragement, he tells funny stories to help you remember the message. One of the funniest stories I've heard on a Sunday morning was his story of waiting for his wife, Victoria, shopping in a souvenir shop at Disneyland. He was talking about staying cool, calm, and collected.

I hope people read this book because I think it will save lives when people learn how important it is to check the condition of their heart with a cardiologist.

In every room in the hospital, there is a sign on the wall close to the beds. It has a picture of six faces. The one on the far left is a smiling face, and the one on the far right is a face with tears. The faces between are gradually looking sadder, going from left to right. Below the faces are a scale of pain: no pain, mild pain, moderate pain, severe pain, and worst possible pain. Written above the faces are the words, "Tell us if you have pain." If you have pain, they give you Percocet or some other painkiller.

The nurses ask you every few hours if you have pain and on what level, on a scale from one to ten. I went through this whole procedure with practically no pain.

I have always been a fairly private person, and it is hard for me to talk about private things, but I have to say this amazing experience has brought me closer to God.

My brother has been religious all his life. He had a calling from God at an early age. He used to hold church services in the tool shed at the back of our home, for the kids in our neighborhood, when he was ten years old. He had me sitting on a wooden crate pounding away on an old fruit case that we used as a pretend organ and singing "Onward Christian Solders."

My brother, The Reverend John Kohler, recently passed away from renal failure. Around six hundred people attended his funeral. He met and befriended many people in this lifetime, including Dame Joan Sutherland and Prince Michael Romanov and his wife, who is related to the last Russian tsar, Nikolai Romanov. Pretty amazing—a kid from the western suburbs of Sydney, Australia, was invited to attend the ceremony a few years ago when they moved the last Russian tsar's mother's body from Germany to St. Petersburg in Russia.

My sister Lilli went to Pakistan when she was in her twenties as a missionary, where she met her Australian husband. I have always believed in God but have not been as religious as them. I always thought I may have been behind the kitchen door when they gave out religion. Our parents always had us going to church as kids, and I used to sing in the church choir.

I have always thought of the glass being half full rather than the glass half empty. I find myself thanking God every day for all I have: my home and loving wife, our children, our dog, and the repaired heart I have.

A nurse in the hospital told me that a Swiss mountain climber, Veronika Meyer, had climbed to the summit of Mt. Everest in 2007. She did this after having mechanical heart valve implant surgery. It is thought she is the first to achieve such a feat. Truly amazing!

Here is a short list of the many well-known people who have had heart valve surgery.

- Barbara Walters
- David Letterman
- Ed Koch
- Jim Lehrer
- Barbara Bush
- Robin Williams
- Arnold Schwarzenegger

The surgery certainly hasn't slowed the first two on this list.

Barbara Walters boasted on her show, *The View*, how her scar was no longer visible and how great she felt. She said people asked her how she felt with a sad look on their face, and she would say, "I feel great!"

David Letterman told Oprah on her show that he loved his open-heart surgery, and all that followed it was good.

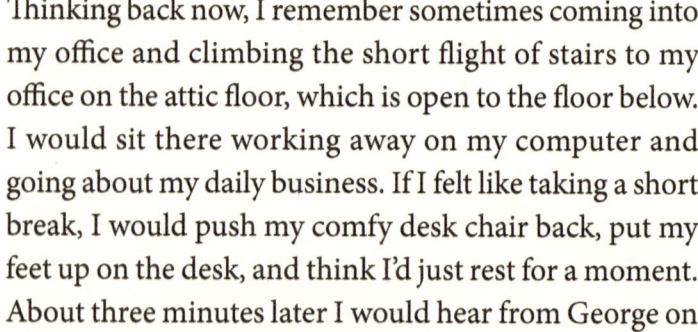

Thinking back now, I remember sometimes coming into my office and climbing the short flight of stairs to my office on the attic floor, which is open to the floor below. I would sit there working away on my computer and going about my daily business. If I felt like taking a short break, I would push my comfy desk chair back, put my feet up on the desk, and think I'd just rest for a moment. About three minutes later I would hear from George on the office floor below. "Hey Roger, wake up."

Great, no more of that now.

George is a very reassuring person. Two years ago, I mentioned I had bought a bicycle and one Sunday afternoon I was going to take a two hour ride on the famous bike trail that stretches some forty miles along picturesque ponds and lakes from Dennis to Wellfleet. He replied "Where shall I send the ambulance".

So now when someone asks, "How are you?"

I reply "I am good, I just had the Audi serviced and I've just had an AVR (aortic valve replacement).

I was scheduled to see Dr. Kalin five weeks after the surgery. He was happy with my progress, and I was taken off the heart rhythm pill, so I was now down to five medications a day.

I mentioned I was thinking of publishing a book about my surgery experience, and he thought it wasn't a bad idea because it could make more people aware of the dangers of heart attack.

I have to say my thoughts go back to Dr. Reagan. In a way I feel he probably saved my life because if it had not been for him I probably would have continued my life unaware I had a major problem. He has been my primary care doctor for only a short time and a week ago he suggested I try muscle relaxers for a back pain problem I have had for fifteen years. It seems they are working and I am a little surprised my doctors over the last fifteen years have not suggested them. I have always been told to take Tylenol, Aleve, Motrin or something similar. These drugs can cause internal bleeding (something I don't need) and have given me almost no relief.

It was Sunday afternoon, and I had turned on the PGA, which was a Sunday afternoon pastime for me. I could smell coffee brewing in the kitchen. "Honey, would you like a piece of cake?" Adele asked.

I was looking at a blue folder that had been sitting on a table in my room from the Beth Israel Deaconess Medical Center. It had writing on the front cover.

We Promise:

To see you every hour.
To attend to your bathroom and hygiene needs.
To ask about your pain.
To keep the call bell and phone within your reach.
Your safety and comfort is important to us.

This was reassuring, and believe me, this is one great hospital. During my stay at the hospital I would have come in contact with at least thirty people, including doctors, nurses and staff and I found everyone pleasant, competent and with a genuine desire to help you. Not one person was unpleasant.

What most people don't know is that *nearly half those who die from heart attacks each year never showed prior symptoms of heart disease.* Right now, millions of people over age forty are suffering from heart disease and do not even know it.

Heart disease is the *number-one killer in America*, and this is true for not only men but women also. In fact, *nearly one-third of all US deaths result from heart disease.*

If the writing of this book saves only one life, then it will have been worth it.

I thought, *If this book gets published, great; if not, then it was fun to write and pass the time during my recovery.*

I attribute my remarkable recovery to Dr. Brian Reagan, Dr. John Kalin, Dr. Kamal Khabbaz, everyone I came in contact with at the Beth Israel Deaconess Medical Center, all my family (especially my loving wife, Adele), and God.

A Remarkable Experience

The End

References

American Heart Association.

\# University of Southern California Keck School of Medicine.

\# www.SimpleHeartTest.com

\# The Patient's Guide to Heart Valve Surgery.

www.ingramcontent.com/pod-product-compliance
Lightning Source LLC
Chambersburg PA
CBHW030407290526
45785CB00004B/1935